The Gi Diet
Shopping and Eating Out Pocket Guide

Rick Gallop

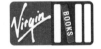

This edition first published in Great Britain in 2004 by:
Virgin Books
Thames Wharf Studios
Rainville Road
London W6 9HA

This edition published by arrangement with Random House Canada,
a division of Random House of Canada Limited

A catalogue record for the book is available from the British Library.

ISBN: 0 7535 0910 5

Designed by Smith & Gilmour, London
Printed and bound by the Bath Press

CONTENTS

Introduction

Over the past couple of years since *The Gi Diet* was launched, I have received hundreds of e-mails requesting a more portable version of the book to use as a guide when shopping and eating out. Though there are removable pages in the original book for both such purposes, readers have seemed reluctant do so in case the pages were misplaced or lost.

The Gi Diet Shopping and Eating Out Pocket Guide is the answer to those e-mail requests and is complementary to and not a replacement for either *The Gi Diet*, or *Living the Gi Diet*. Without reading and understanding the principles of the G.I. Diet, this guide will make little sense. So, if this book is your first introduction to the G.I. Diet, then I suggest you purchase either *The Gi Diet*, or its companion recipe book *Living the Gi Diet*.

In this guide, you will find all the information you need regarding what foods you should shop for and what to choose when you are eating in a restaurant or café. I have also included practical tips to help you make better decisions about what you buy.

Shopping the G.I. Diet way should not be more expensive than your current budget. Fresh vegetables and fruit in season are always good value. Out of season, frozen vegetables and fruits are just as nutritious and can be relatively inexpensive, if bought in bulk. Most supermarkets now have a terrific selection of large bags of frozen fruits and vegetables at great prices.

Try not to go for canned products, as the canning process requires the food to be treated at high temperatures to avoid spoilage, which both reduces the nutritional value and increases the food's G.I. rating. So, for preference, buy canned products only when fresh, dried, or frozen, ones are not available.

In fact, because you will be buying far less processed foods than before, you should make substantial savings, since any processing by the manufacturer simply provides a reason to charge considerably more than the cost of the original unprocessed product.

In the following pages, you will find advice on how to pick the best cuts of meat and poultry, or the best seafood, as well as how to read food labels so that you know what you are really buying. Plus, there are lists of which foods fall into the green-, yellow- and red-light categories and the ultimate G.I. Diet Shopping List.

Eating out should always be a pleasant experience, but when you are on a diet it can become a bit of a minefield and you don't want to have to put your social life on hold just because you are on a diet. It is inevitable that some cuisines should be completely avoided during Phase 1 of the G.I. Diet, but it is handy to know what to choose when you are faced with a highly tempting menu and what to do even when you have reached Phase 2 and are maintaining your weight loss.

The emphasis in this guide is on convenience and practicality, taking into account the realities of the world we live in. I hope you will find it helpful in making the right choices when faced with the vast range of choices and brands in today's supermarkets, restaurants and fast-food outlets.

As always, your feedback is extremely valuable, so that others can benefit from your experiences. I can be reached through my website at www.gidiet.co.uk

Shopping Guide

One thing you should never do is to go shopping on an empty stomach. In the temple of temptation, the supermarket, you could easily be driven by your tummy to give way to cravings and finish up with a shopping cart that is distinctly not green light!

If you are just starting the G.I. Diet, make sure you clear out your pantry, fridge and freezer of all red-light foods. Don't waste them: give them to the local food bank, homeless shelter or your neighbours.

Further on you will find lists of green-light and yellow-light foods. Remember that yellow-light foods should be reserved for Phase 2 when you have reached your desired target weight. But before you look at the food lists, here is a guide to reading labels, which contains information that you should bear in mind when you are making your choices.

READING LABELS

Although most of the foods listed are the generic categories (e.g. 'Pasta' rather than 'Barilla Pasta'), the reality is that most of us buy brands not categories, unless we're shopping in bulk food sections or stores. Obviously, I could not hope to list the thousands of brands available, so when trying to determine which brand is your best green-light choice, read the label. If you can't find the nutritional information on the package, then you may reasonably surmise that the manufacturer has something to hide.

Here are a few tips when trying to decipher labelling information:

NUTRITIONAL FACTS

NUTRITION INFORMATION
TYPICAL VALUES PER ½ PACKET

Energy 1237kJ/298kcal

Protein 8.9g, Carbohydrate
17.5g, of which sugars 4.2g,
Fat 21.3g, of which saturates
4.4g, Fibre 1.6g, Sodium 0.1g.

TYPICAL VALUES PER 100G

Energy 2474kJ/595kcal

Protein 17.8g, Carbohydrate
35.0g, of which sugars 8.4g,
Fat 42.6g, of which saturates
8.8g, Fibre 3.2g, Sodium 0.2g.

The ingredients that are critical in making the right green-light choices are:

Serving Size
Is the serving size realistic, or has the manufacturer lowered it (often the case with cold cereals) so that the calorie and fat totals in particular look better than their competition? Also, when comparing one brand to another in any category, make sure you are comparing the same serving sizes.

Calories
One of the key criteria for green-light foods is their calorie density. Again, when comparing brands, this is the first item to check and it is often a warning flag for fat and sugar levels.

Fat

Here we want to check both the fat and, more importantly, the saturated fat levels. To the government's credit, they have included Trans (trans fatty acids), which are the worst of the saturated fats. Interestingly, even the US has yet to include trans fatty acids in their labelling regulations. Combine both numbers to come up with the total saturated fat content.

Fibre

This is a critical component of the G.I. Diet, as the G.I. of the food is significantly affected by its fibre content. Fibrous foods have a lower G.I., so when comparing brands go for fibre as a key ingredient.

The other ingredients such as cholesterol and sodium are less of an issue, unless you have a medical problem, such as heart disease, stroke, or hypertension (high blood pressure).

BREAD

The product with the most confusing labelling statements is bread – I use the word 'confusing' charitably, as others might call it 'misleading'. Things are not always what they seem to be. Beware of descriptions such as 'enriched flour', or 'unbleached flour' which is actually white flour where all the nutrients found in the wheat germ and bran have been stripped away. 'Enriched' indicates that a few minerals and vitamins have been added back.

So don't be misled by fancy descriptions such as 'multigrain', 'whole grains', or '12 grains' where in fact there is likely to be more sugar than whole grain.

So what should you do? The answer is to look for '100% wholemeal' or 'wholemeal bread', preferably 'stone milled'. Stone-milled flour is coarser than the flour produced by today's steel rollers and has a lower G.I.

Whatever your choice of grain, the critical factor is fibre. Look for a minimum of 5 to 6 g per two-slice serving.

Sugar

Sugar levels are something to be aware of in certain brands where the manufacturer may be trumpeting the low-fat characteristics of the product while quietly bumping up the sugar content to offset any perceived taste shortfall. Yoghurts, cereals and ice cream are good examples of this practice.

Best Green-light Buy

To recap, when looking for the best green-light buy, choose the ones with the following nutritional characteristics

- Lower calories
- Lower fat – particularly the combination of saturated fat and trans fat
- Higher fibre

SHOPPING LIST

Meat, Poultry and Fish

Most meats contain fat especially saturated (bad) fat, so it's important both to select meats that have had all the visible fat trimmed and that are intrinsically lean. Simply trimming visible fat can reduce the fat content by an average of 50 per cent. The traditional benchmark for lean meat is skinless chicken breast. Veal is the low-fat standard for non-poultry meats.

Remember: the recommended serving size is 4 oz (120 g).

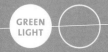

BEEF

Top round steak
Eye round Steak
Extra lean ground

LAMB

PORK

Deli ham

Back bacon

BEEF

Sirloin tip
Sirloin steak
Lean ground

LAMB

Fore shank
Leg shank
Centre cut
Loin chop

PORK

Tenderloin

Centre loin chop
Boiled ham

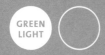

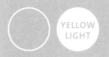

VEAL
Cutlet
Rib roast
Blade steak

CHICKEN/TURKEY
(SKINLESS)
Breast
Leg
(Also lean deli cuts of
cooked chicken or turkey)

FISH/SEAFOOD
All fish is green light
and delicious, but DO
NOT choose any fish
which has been breaded
or partially cooked in
batter ready for final
baking or frying.

STOCK LIST

Here is a guide to what you should buy to keep in stock generally.

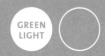

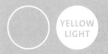

Larder/Pantry

BAKING/COOKING

Baking powder/soda
Cocoa
Dried beans (all)
Raisins*
Sliced almonds
Wheat/oat bran
Wholemeal flour

BAKING/COOKING

Dried Apricots
Dried Cranberries

* acceptable as a baking ingredient

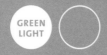

BEANS (LEGUMES)

Black

Black eyed

Butter

Chickpeas

Haricot/Navy

Italian

Kidney

Lentils

Lima

Mung

Pigeon

Pinto

Romano

Soy

Split

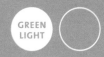

GREEN LIGHT

BEANS (TINNED)
Baked beans (low-fat)
Mixed salad beans
Most varieties
Vegetarian chili

BREAD
100% stone-ground
wholemeal
Whole grain with
2.5 to 3 g fibre per slice

CEREALS (BREAKFAST)
All bran
Bran Buds
Fibre 1
100% Bran
Porridge oats
(traditional large flake)
Soya protein powder

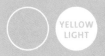

YELLOW LIGHT

BEANS (TINNED)

BREAD
Pita (wholemeal)

CEREALS (BREAKFAST)
Shredded Wheat Bran

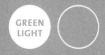

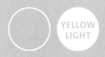

GREEN LIGHT

**DRESSINGS/
FAT/OILS/NUTS**

Almonds
Cashews
Hazelnuts
Macadamia
Margarine
(low-fat/light)
Mayonnaise (no-fat)
Olive oil
Pistachio
Rapeseed oil
Salad dressings
(no-fat/low sugar)
Vegetable oil spray

YELLOW LIGHT

**DRESSINGS/
FAT/OILS/NUTS**

Corn oil
Mayonnaise (light)
Peanuts
Peanut oil
Pecans
Salad dressings (light)
Sesame oil
Sunflower oil
Walnuts

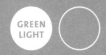

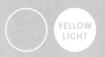

DRINKS

Bottled water
(unsweetened)
Chocolate (light)
Coffee (decaf)
Diet soft drinks
(no caffeine)
Herbal teas
Tea
Tonic water

DRINKS

Fruit juices
Red wine

FRUITS (FRESH)

Apples	Limes
Blackberries	Nectarines
Blueberries	Oranges
Cherries	Peaches
Grapefruit	Pears
Grapes	Plums
Guavas	Raspberries
Lemons	Strawberries

FRUITS (FRESH)

Apricots
Bananas
Kiwi
Mangos
Papaya
Pineapple

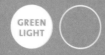

GREEN LIGHT

**FRUIT
(TINNED/BOTTLED)**
Apple sauce (no sugar)
(e.g. Clearspring
Organic Apple Purée)
Mandarin oranges
Peaches in juice or water
Pears in juice or water

GRAINS
Amaranth
Barley
Buckwheat
Bulgar
Kasha (toasted
buckwheat)
Millet
Rice (basmati, wild,
brown, long grain)
Soya protein powder
Wheat grain

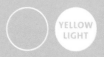

YELLOW LIGHT

**FRUIT
(TINNED/BOTTLED)**
Fruit cocktail
(in juice)

GRAINS
Corn

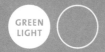 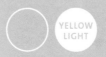

PASTA

Capellini
Cellophane Noodles
(Mung bean)
Fettuccine
Linguine
Macaroni
Penne
Rigatoni
Spaghetti
Vermicelli

PASTA SAUCES

Light sauces with or
without vegetables
(with no added sugar)

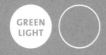

SEASONINGS/ CONDIMENTS
Chilli powder
Extracts (vanilla etc)
Flavoured vinegars/ sauces
Garlic
Herbs
Horseradish
Hummus
Lemon/lime juice
Mustard
Pepper (all types)
Salsa (low sugar
Soy sauce
(low sodium)
Spices
Teriyaki sauce
Worcestershire
sauce

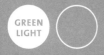

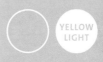

GREEN LIGHT

SNACKS
Canned fruits
Dairy (see Fridge/Freezer)
Food bars (12-15 g protein;
4-5 g fat) e.g. Myoplex /
Power Protein
Fresh fruit (see list)
Fresh vegetables (see list)
Nuts (see fats and oils)

SOUPS
Baxter's Healthy Choice
(Vegetable or
bean-based only)

YELLOW LIGHT

SNACKS
Bananas
Dark chocolate (70% cocoa)
Popcorn (light
microwaveable)

SOUPS
Tinned chicken noodle
Tinned lentil
Tinned tomato

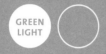

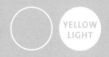

VEGETABLES

Alfalfa sprouts
Asparagus
Aubergine
Beans
(green or runner)
Bok choy
Broccoli
Brussel sprouts
Cabbage
Capers
Carrots
Cauliflower
Celery
Collard greens
Courgettes
Cucumber
Lettuce
Mangetout
Mushrooms
Mustard greens
Okra

VEGETABLES

Artichokes
Beets
Corn
Pumpkin
Squash
Sweet potatoes
Yams

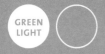

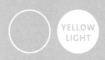

Olives
Onions
Parsley
Peas
Peppers
Peppers (chilis)
Pickles
Potatoes (new only)
Radicchio
Radishes
Sauerkraut
Scallions
Sugar snap peas
Swiss Chard
Spinach
Tomatoes

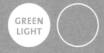

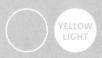

Fridge/Freezer

DAIRY

Buttermilk
Cheese (Fat-free)
Cottage cheese (low-fat
or fat-free)
Ice cream (low fat
and no added sugar)
Milk (skimmed)
Sour cream (low-fat or
fat-free)
Yoghurt (no fat/no sugar)

DAIRY

Cream cheese (light)
Frozen yoghurt (low
fat/sugar)
Ice cream (low fat)
Milk (semi skimmed)
Soft Margarine (non
hydrogenated)
Sour cream (light)
Yoghurt (low fat)

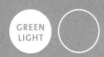

GREEN LIGHT

**MEAT/POULTRY/
FISH/EGGS**
(See lists on pages 16–17)
Egg whites
Sashimi
Tofu (low fat)

SWEETENERS
Hermesetas Gold
Splenda
Stevia (see page 94)

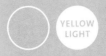

YELLOW LIGHT

**MEAT/POULTRY/
FISH/EGGS**
See lists on pages 16–17)
Whole Omega- 3 eggs

Eating Out

Eating out on the G.I. diet is not difficult. Today's restaurants' trend towards the use of vegetable oils, especially olive oil, plus a greater emphasis on grilling rather than frying, a better variety of vegetables, increased salad options and more fish dishes, makes it even easier to dine out the green-light way.

As dining out is often a social occasion, you want to be able to enjoy yourself with your friends and not feel that you are a damper on the occasion. So here are my top 10 suggestions:

1. Just before you go out, have a small bowl of high-fibre cold cereal (such as All Bran) with skimmed milk and sweetener. I often add a couple of spoons of no fat/sugar fruit yoghurt. This will take the edge off your appetite and get some fibre into your tummy, which will help reduce the G.I. of your forthcoming meal.

2. On arrival, drink a glass of water because it will help you feel fuller. A glass of red wine is a good idea, but wait until the main course before drinking.

3. Once the habitual basket of rolls or bread has been passed round, which you should ignore, ask the waiter to remove it (if it's left on the table), as the longer it sits there the more tempted you will be to dig in.

4. If you are having the traditional three courses, opt for a soup or salad first. For soups go for vegetable- or bean-based ones, the chunkier the better. Avoid any that are cream based. For salads, the golden rule is to ask for the dressing on the side because you will only use a fraction of what the restaurant is likely to smother on. And do avoid Caesar salads which come already dressed.

5. If boiled new potatoes are not available and you can't be sure what type of rice is being served, ask to have two other vegetables instead. I have yet to find a restaurant that won't willingly oblige.

6. Stick with low fat cuts of meat (see Shopping List pages 16–17), or poultry where, if necessary, you can remove the skin. Fish and shellfish are an excellent choice but must not be breaded or battered. Remember: as servings tend to be generous in restaurants eat only 120-180g (4–6 oz) (about the size of a pack of cards) and leave the rest.

7. As with salads, ask for any sauces to be put on the side.

8. Puddings/Desserts. This is a real minefield with usually not a lot of green-light choices. If available, fresh fruit and berries without any ice cream, are your best choice. Most other choices are a dietary disaster.

My best advice is to try and avoid dessert. If social pressure becomes overwhelming, or it is a special occasion, ask for extra forks so the dessert can be shared. A couple of forkfuls or so along with your coffee should get you off the hook with minimal damage!

9. Only order decaffeinated coffee. Skimmed decaf cappuccino is our family's favourite choice.

10. Finally, and perhaps most importantly, eat slowly. In the eighteenth century the famous Dr Johnson advocated chewing food 32 times before swallowing! That's going a little overboard, but at least put your fork down between mouthfuls.

The stomach can take between 20 to 30 minutes to let the brain know it feels full. So if you eat quickly, you may be shovelling in more food than you require until your brain says stop. You will also have more time to savour your meal.

SUMMARY

1. Bowl of bran cereal before going out.

2. Drink water on arrival – red wine later with the main course.

3. Ask for the bread basket to be taken away from the table.

4. Choose a soup or salad for the first course, preferably a vegetable/bean soup and not cream based. Ask for salad dressings to be served separately.

5. Two vegetables in lieu of potatoes/rice.

6. Poultry, veal and seafood are the best choices for the main course. Never choose fried food.

7. All sauces should be served on the side.

8. Desserts: avoid or ask for extra forks. Choose fresh fruit/berries, if available.

9. Choose decaffeinated coffee

10. Eat slowly

All You Can Eat Buffets

These can be your best or worst option depending on your self-control. Best because you are free to make your own selection and it's hard not to come away with a green-light plate. Worst because of the temptations to have a little bit of everything and wish you had chosen the larger plate! If you're like me, by the time you are halfway round the buffet table, your plate is already full and you try to pile on those tantalising foods that you wished you had seen earlier.

The secret is to do a quick reconnaissance of the whole buffet before picking up your plate and starting. Just follow the green-light ground rules, scope out the options and the buffet will you be your best dining option bar none.

International Cuisine

One of my favourite activities when dining out is trying foods from other countries. Here are a few extra tips when you dine on some of the popular international cuisines such as Italian, Greek, Chinese, Asian and Indian.

ITALIAN

Not surprisingly, we immediately think of pasta as the archetypal Italian dish and generally we tend to overdo our servings compared with those you would find in restaurants in Italy. There it is normally served as an appetiser and that is really what you should try and eat it as, or as a side dish to a main course. If you do choose it as a side dish, then ask for half a portion. Also, try and choose wholemeal pasta, if possible. Under no circumstances should pasta form the base of the meal as has become commonplace in countries other than Italy.

The serving should not exceed one quarter of the plate (half a cricket ball). Choose a main dish of meat or fish (veal is popular in Italian restaurants and a great choice with its low saturated fat content) and lots of fresh vegetables. And forget the tiramisu and ice cream – both Italian specialities – for dessert.

GREEK

The classic Souvlaki (chicken, lamb, beef or pork) with rice and salad is by far your best choice. Often potatoes are also served with the rice so ask for an extra vegetable in lieu of the potatoes.

Salads can be a problem, if the chef is heavy handed with the feta cheese. Ask if you can have the feta and the dressing on the side. Avoid the gyros, dolmades, and moussaka as they are full of saturated fat.

Greek deserts, delicious as they are, are a calorie disaster especially the popular baklava. If it's too much temptation, ask for a couple of forks and share it with your eating companions.

CHINESE

It is a real challenge to follow the G.I. Diet when eating out at Chinese restaurants. Given the low-fibre nature of much of the prepared food, it's not surprising you can eat a large Chinese meal and be hungry and/or asleep an hour later. However, with some effort it can be done. Look for dishes containing steamed or stir-fried vegetables that have had their flavour enhanced by oyster sauce, garlic and ginger.

Since much Chinese cooking rests on beds of rice or noodles you need to pay attention to both the type and the amount. Most of the rice used is short grain which has a glutinous sticky surface and is classified as red light. You may be lucky if you ask for basmati, wild, or long-grain rice instead. For noodles look for 'cellophane noodles' made from dried mung beans. All other noodles are red light. Keep the portion of noodles or rice to no more than a quarter of your plate – it's too easy to heap it up!

Stick with savoury sauces and avoid sweet sauces.

Eat lots of steamed vegetables and avoid fried meat or fish, especially when they are incorporated in dumplings. Unfortunately, there is little you can to about some of the hidden health risks, such as the high sodium levels in many sauces and the frequent use of saturated and trans fat oils used in cooking the dishes.

You can eat Chinese the green-light way if you cook at home. However, if needs must, then dine out carefully and only occasionally. There are better alternatives around.

SOUTH ASIAN/INDIAN

Fruit, vegetables, legumes, and whole grains are predominant in Indian cuisine. Many South Asians are vegetarians and use lentils and beans as their protein source. Helpings of meat or fish tend to be modest. Basmati and long grain rice are extensively used. All this makes Indian restaurants an excellent green-light choice for dining out.

The most significant danger to your health and waistline is in the food preparation. Frying, often deep-fat frying is commonplace and to make things worse, 'ghee' (clarified butter), a highly saturated fat, is frequently used. So make sure you ask how the food is prepared. Baked or grilled dishes are your best options. Similarly, dairy products, such as yogurt, are usually full fat and should be consumed in small quantities.

One food to watch is bread. Whereas in India the South favours rice and the North bread, here we tend to use ample quantities of both. As when dining out anywhere, avoid bread. If unavoidable, choose wholemeal baked chapatti.

Many restaurants offer heaped dishes of coconut slices, raisins and sweeteners. These are red light. Similarly be careful of the fruits. Mangos, papayas and custard apples are yellow light; guavas however are green light.

By exercising some caution and restraint, eating the Indian way can be an excellent G.I. Diet experience.

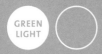

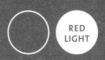

EATING OUT SUMMARY TABLE

BREAKFAST
All-Bran
Back bacon
Egg Whites – Omelette
Egg Whites – Scrambled
Fruit
Porridge oats
Wholemeal toast
(one slice)
Yoghurt (low-fat)

BREAKFAST
Cold cereals
Bacon/sausage
Eggs
Scones
Pancakes/waffles

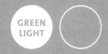

GREEN LIGHT

LUNCH

Fast food (see opposite)
Meats – deli style ham/
chicken/turkey breast
Pasta – ¼ plate maximum
Salads – low-fat
(dressing on the side)
Sandwiches –
open-faced/wholemeal
Soups –
chunky vegetable
and bean
Vegetables
Wraps – ½ wholemeal
pita, no mayonnaise

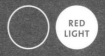

RED LIGHT

LUNCH

Bakery products
Butter/mayonnaise
Cheese
Fast food (see page 49)
Pasta-based meals
Pizza/bread/bagels
Potatoes (replace with
double vegetables)

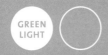

GREEN LIGHT

DINNER
Beef/lamb/pork
(see page 16)*
Chicken/turkey (no skin)
Fruit
Pasta – ¼ plate
Rice (basmati, brown,
wild, long grain) –
¼ plate
Salads – low-fat
(dressing on the side)
Seafood –
not breaded or battered
Soups –
chunky vegetable
and bean
Veal
Vegetables

*Yellow light

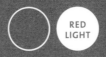

RED LIGHT

DINNER
Beef/lamb/pork
Bread
Butter/mayonnaise
Caesar salad
Potatoes (replace with
double vegetables)
Puddings
Soups – cream based

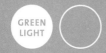

SNACKS
Almonds
Food bar – ½
Fresh fruit
Hazelnuts
Yoghurt – no fat/no sugar

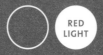

SNACKS
Chips, all types
Biscuits/Cakes/Scones
Popcorn, regular

PORTIONS

Meat –
Palm of hand /
Pack of cards
Rice/pasta –
Maximum ¼ plate
Vegetables –
Minimum ½ plate

Fast Food

A couple of years ago the idea of getting a green-light meal at a fast food restaurant was simply laughable. Well, partly due to the threat of legal action and a stagnant market share, the major fast food chains are finally offering some healthy options. In all fairness, Subway has pioneered the move to healthy choices for some time now, which has been reflected in their successful growth. They have replaced McDonald's in the United States as the number one fast food chain and are expanding rapidly in the United Kingdom.

The problem with most fast food outlets is the quality and quantity of the food. Hamburgers are soaked in saturated fat; fish and chicken are coated in deep-fried batter or breading. And all the trimmings – chips, ketchup, shakes and fizzy drinks – are all loaded with fat and sugar. To compound it all, everything is super-sized. Food is a relatively cheap commodity in this country so doubling the hamburger, fizzy drink or chips for a few pennies more is an attractive enticement to make this dietary disaster even worse. No wonder our kids are setting obesity records and becoming diabetics. So what are the points of light in this sea of gloom? Let's deal with each of the major outlets in turn.

NOTE. Always eat burgers (called sandwiches in the trade) open faced and throwaway the top half of the bun. Always ask for low-fat dressings.

McDonald's

McDonald's is the grandfather (or godfather?) of the fast food industry with the largest worldwide sales. With products such as the quarter-pounder and large fries weighing in at 970 calories and 47 g of fat, they have not surprisingly become the favourite target for nutritionists and other health activists.

McDonald's has made a tentative start to changing their menu, but the healthy options are still only a nominal part of the dishes on offer. Here are your best options:

GREEN LIGHT	YELLOW LIGHT
SALADS	**SALADS**
Pasta Salad with Chicken	Caesar Salad with Chicken
SNACK	**SNACK**
Strawberry Yogurt Burst	Classic Chicken

Burger King

Burger King is the last of the major burger chains to enter the lower fat market. Still, better late than never, and I hope they'll be encouraged to broaden their offerings. Suffice to say that with their flagship Whopper and fries weighing in at 1117 calories with a mind and artery numbing 58 g of fat, they clearly have a lot to make up for.

GREEN LIGHT	YELLOW LIGHT
SALAD	**SANDWICHES**
Flame Grilled Chicken Salad	Chicken Whopper Lite

Subway

Subway is to be congratulated as the pacesetter in the fast food industry with its broad range of low-fat products. The company deserves a G.I. Diet gold star and warrants your support.

GREEN LIGHT	GREEN LIGHT
SANDWICHES	**SOUPS**
(6 IN UNDER 6 G SUBS)	Chicken and rice
Roast beef	Creole chicken gumbo
Roast chicken breast	Minestrone
Subway club	Roasted chicken noodle
Turkey breast	Tomato Garden vegetable
Turkey breast and ham	Vegetable beef
Veggie Delite	Vegetarian vegetable

GREEN LIGHT	YELLOW LIGHT
DELI SUBS	**DELI SUBS**
Ham Deli	Tuna deli
Roast Beef Deli	
Turkey Breast Deli	

Note: the best choices in 6-inch rolls are Italian or Wheat. Remember to eat open faced.

GREEN LIGHT	YELLOW LIGHT
SALADS	
Ham	Roasted Chicken
Roast Beef	
Subway Club	
Turkey breast and ham	
Veggie Delite	

DRESSINGS:
Fat-free Honey Mustard;
Fat-free Wine Vinaigrette;
Fat-free Sweet Onion.

Other Fast Food

From here it is downhill. Few pizza outlets offer anything which is remotely green light and even the popular Pizza Express's Salad Nicoise, where you might expect a glimmer of green light, has a numbing 49 g of fat (your entire daily fat intake) and 827 calories!

Similarly, fast food outlets, such as KFC where all the food is breaded and deep fried, have no options that can be listed as green or even yellow light. They are for very rare occasions once you have moved into Phase 2 of the G.I. Diet.

Sandwich shops are little better. Prêt a Manger is a fat lover's heaven and unconditionally red light.

This information was correct at time of going to press. However, as this is a dynamic field, you may wish to check the menus or websites of the outlets mentioned from time to time to see if they have expanded their green-light menus.

Takeaway Food

The best advice is don't opt for takeaway food. The emphasis for these food outlets is on price, convenience, speed and not nutrition. If you must choose a takeaway option, then Indian is your best bet.

FISH AND CHIPS

The UK's most famous contribution to international cuisine and obesity, the traditional fish in batter and accompanying chips are a classic example of taking an ideal food, fish, and adulterating it with the calorie-loaded batter and deep frying it in oil. Throw in those deep-fried potatoes and you have the making of a nutritional disaster.

CHINESE

Not a good choice though there are a few opportunities (see page 41).

INDIAN

Probably your best choice (see page 43).

PIZZA

A no-no for people in Phase I and, sadly, it should only be a special treat for people in Phase 2.

The G.I. Diet Food Guide

This chart lists every food you can think of in one of three categories based on the colours of a traffic light. Foods listed in the red-light or 'stop' category are high-G.I., high-calorie foods that should be avoided. Some of these may surprise you, for example, melba toast, mashed potatoes, turnip and watermelon are all red-light. Your body digests them so quickly that you are hungry again an hour later. Foods in the yellow-light or 'caution' category – for example, sourdough bread, corn and bananas – have moderate G.I. ratings, but they do raise insulin levels to the point where weight loss is not going to happen. Foods in the green-light or 'go ahead' category are the ones that will allow you to lose weight. Chicken, long-grain rice and asparagus are all green-light foods. Eat them and watch your weight drop.

RED

BEANS

Baked beans with pork
Broad
Refried beans

YELLOW

GREEN

BEANS

Black
Black eyed
Butter
Chickpeas
Haricot/Navy
Italian
Kidney
Lentils

Lima
Mung
Pigeon
Pinto
Romano
Soy
Split

BEANS (TINNED)

Baked beans (low-fat)
Mixed salad beans
Most varieties
Vegetarian chili

BEVERAGES

Alcoholic drinks*
Fruit drinks
Milk (whole)
Regular coffee
Regular soft drinks
Sweetened juice

*In Phase II a glass of wine and the
occasional beer may be included

BEVERAGES

Diet soft drinks (caffeinated)
Milk (semi-skimmed)
Red wine*
Regular coffee
(with skimmed milk, no sugar)
Unsweetened fruit juices:
Apple
Cranberry
Grapefruit
Orange
Pear
Pineapple

BEVERAGES

Bottled water
Tonic water
Decaffeinated coffee
(with skimmed milk,
no sugar)
Diet soft drinks (no caffeine)
Herbal teas
Light instant chocolate
Milk (skimmed)
Tea (with skimmed
milk, no sugar)

RED

BREADS

Bagels
Baguette/Croissants
Cereal/Granola bars
Crispbreads
Doughnuts
Hamburger buns
Hot dog buns
Kaiser rolls
Melba toast
Muffins
Pancakes/Waffles
Pizza
Stuffing
Tortillas
White bread

YELLOW

BREADS

Pita (wholemeal)
Whole grain breads

GREEN

BREADS

100% stone-ground
wholemeal*
Homemade muffins
(see Living the Gi Diet
p. 167–169)
Homemade pancakes
(see Living the Gi Diet
pp. 104 and 106)
Whole grain, high-fibre
breads (2½ to 3g of fibre
per slice)*

* Limit quantity
* Use a single slice only per serving

CEREALS

All cold cereals
except those listed
as yellow –
or green-light
Granola
Muesli (commercial)

CEREALS

Shredded Wheat Bran

CEREALS

All-Bran
Bran Buds
Fibre First
High Fibre Bran/Alpen
Homemade Muesli
(see *Living the Gi Diet* p.115)
Oat bran
Porridge oats
(traditional large-flake)
100% Bran
Soya Protein Powder

RED

CEREAL GRAINS

Couscous
Rice (short grain, white, instant)
Rice cakes
Croutons

YELLOW

CEREAL GRAINS

Corn

GREEN

CEREAL GRAINS

Amaranth
Barley
Buckwheat
Bulgar
Kasha (toasted buckwheat)
Millet
Rice (basmati, wild, brown, long grain)
Soya Protein Powder
Wheatgrain

CONDIMENTS/SEASONINGS

Ketchup
Mayonnaise
Tartar sauce

CONDIMENTS/SEASONINGS

Chili powder
Extracts (Vanilla etc)
Flavoured vigegars/sauces
Garlic
Herbs/Spices
Horseradish
Hummus
Lemon/lime juice
Mayonnaise (fat free)
Lemon/lime juice
Mustard
Peppers (all types)
Salsa (low sugar)
Soy sauce (low sodium)
Teriyaki sauce
Worcestershire sauce

RED

DAIRY

Cheese
Chocolate milk
Cottage cheese (regular)
Cream
Cream cheese
Milk (whole)
Sour cream
Yoghurt (regular)

YELLOW

DAIRY

Cheese (low fat)
Cream cheese (light)
Ice cream (low fat)
Milk (semi-skimmed)
Frozen yoghurt
(low fat, low sugar)
Soft margarine
(non-hydrogenated)
Sour cream (light)
Yoghurt (low fat)
Creme fraiche (low fat)

GREEN

DAIRY

Buttermilk
Cheese (fat free)
Cottage cheese
(low fat or fat free)
Fruit yoghurt
(no fat/no sugar)
Ice cream
(low fat and no added
sugar, e.g. Wall's Too Good
to be True)
Milk (skimmed)
Sour cream (fat-free)

FATS AND OILS

Butter
Coconut oil
Hard margarine
Lard
Mayonnaise
Palm oil
Peanut butter
(all varieties)
Salad dressings (regular)
Tropical oils
Vegetable shortening

FATS AND OILS

Corn oil
Mayonnaise (light)
Most nuts
Peanut oil
Peanuts
Pecans
Salad dressings (light)
Sesame oil
Soft margarine
(non-hydrogenated)
Sunflower oil
Vegetable oils
Walnuts

FATS AND OILS

Almonds*
Canola oil*/rapeseed oil
Cashew nuts
Flax seed
Hazelnuts*
Macadamia nuts*
Mayonnaise (fat free)
Olive oil*
Pistachio nuts
Salad dressings (fat free)
Soft margarine (non-
hydrogenated, light)*
Vegetable oil sprays

Limit quantity

RED

FRUITS – FRESH

Cantaloupe
Dates
Honeydew melon
Raisins
Watermelon

YELLOW

FRUITS – FRESH

Apricots (fresh)
Bananas
Kiwi
Mangos
Papaya
Pineapple

GREEN

FRUITS – FRESH

Apples
Blackberries
Blueberries
Cherries
Grapefruit
Grapes
Guavas
Lemons
Limes
Oranges
Nectarines
Peaches
Pears
Plums
Raspberries
Strawberries

FRUITS – BOTTLED, TINNED, FROZEN, DRIED

All tinned fruit in syrup

Apple sauce containing sugar

Most dried fruit*

For baking, it is okay to use a modest amount of dried fruit

FRUITS – BOTTLED, TINNED, FROZEN, DRIED

Dried apricots

Dried cranberries

Fruit cocktail in juice

FRUITS – BOTTLED, TINNED, FROZEN, DRIED

Apple sauce (no sugar)
e.g. Clearspring Organic

Apple Purée

Frozen berries

Mandarin oranges

Peaches in juice or water

Pears in juice or water

RED

FRUIT JUICES**

Fruit drinks
Sweetened juices
Prune
Watermelon

Whenever possible eat the fruit rather than drink its juice

MEAT, POULTRY, FISH, EGGS AND SOY

Minced beef
(more than 10% fat)
Hamburgers
Hot dogs
Processed meats

YELLOW

FRUIT JUICES**

Apple (unsweetened)
Cranberry (unsweetened)
Grapefruit (unsweetened)
Orange (unsweetened)
Pear (unsweetened)
Pineapple (unsweetened)

MEAT, POULTRY, FISH, EGGS AND SOY

Minced beef (lean)
Sirloin tip
Sirloin steak
Lamb (Tenderloin,
Centre loin chop, Boiled ham)

GREEN

FRUIT JUICES**

MEAT, POULTRY, FISH, EGGS AND SOY

All seafood, fresh,
frozen or tinned***
Back bacon
Beef (Top round steak,
Eye round steak)

MEAT, POULTRY, FISH, EGGS AND SOY (CONT)

Regular bacon

Sausages

Whole regular eggs

Sushi (it's the rice)

MEAT, POULTRY, FISH, EGGS AND SOY (CONT)

Pork (Fore shank, Leg shank, Centre cut, Loin chop)

Turkey bacon

Whole omega-3 eggs (e.g. Columbus)

MEAT, POULTRY, FISH, EGGS AND SOY (CONT)

Chicken breast (skinless)

Egg whites

Lean deli ham

Minced beef (extra lean)

Quorn**

Sashimi

Soy/whey protein powder

Tofu

Turkey breast (skinless), leg

Veal (Cutlet, Rib Roast, Blade steak)

** Possible health risk
(see www.cspinet.org)

*** Avoid breaded or battered seafood

GREEN

PASTA*

Capellini
Cellophane noodles
(mung bean)
Fettuccine
Linguine
Macaroni
Penne
Rigatoni
Spaghetti
Vermicelli

YELLOW

RED

PASTA*

All tinned pastas
Gnocchi
Macaroni and cheese
Noodles (tinned
or instant)
Pasta filled with with
cheese or meat

Try to use wholemeal or protein-enriched pasta

PASTA SAUCES

Alfredo
Sauces with added
meat or cheese
Sauces with added
sugar or sucrose

SNACKS

Bagels
Bread
Chocolates and sweets
Cookies
Biscuits
Doughnuts
French fries
Ice cream
Jelly (all varieties)
Muffins (commercial)
Popcorn (regular)

PASTA SAUCES

Sauces with
vegetables (no added sugar)

SNACKS

Bananas
Dark chocolate (70% cocoa)*
Ice cream (low fat and no
added sugar)
Most nuts*
Popcorn (light, microwaveable)

Limit quantity (see page 77)

PASTA SAUCES

Light sauces with
or without vegetables
(no added sugar)

SNACKS

Almonds*
Apple sauce (unsweetened)
Tinned peaches/pears
in juice or water
Canned fruits
Cottage cheese (1% or fat-free
protein)
Food bars (12–15g protein;
4–5g fat) e.g. Myoplex/
Power Protein (see Living
the Gi Diet p.176)
Nuts (see fats and oils)

RED

SNACKS (CONT)

Crisps/Pretzels

Raisins

Rice cakes

Sorbet

Tortilla chips

Mixed dried fruit
and nuts

YELLOW

SNACKS (CONT)

GREEN

SNACKS (CONT)

Fruit yoghurt (fat and
sugar free)

Ice cream (low fat and
no added sugar, e.g. Wall's
Too Good to be True)

Hazelnuts*

Homemade muffins
(see *Living the Gi Diet* p. 240)

Most fresh fruit

Most fresh vegetables

Soy nuts*

* Limit quantity (see page 77)

SOUPS

All cream-based soups
Tinned black bean
Tinned green pea
Puréed vegetable
Tinned split pea

SUGAR AND SWEETENERS**

Corn syrup
Glucose
Honey
Molasses
Sugar (all types)
Treacle

SOUPS

Tinned chicken noodle
Tinned lentil
Tinned tomato

SUGAR AND SWEETENERS**

Fructose

SOUPS

All homemade soups made with green-light ingredients.
Chunky bean and vegetabe soups (e.g. Baxter's Healthy Choice)

SUGAR AND SWEETENERS**

Aspartame
Hermesetas Gold
Splenda
Stevia

RED

VEGETABLES

Broad beans
French fries
Hash browns
Parsnips
Potatoes (instant)
Potatoes (mashed
or baked)
Swede
Turnip

YELLOW

VEGETABLES

Artichokes
Beets
Corn
Avocado (¼ per serving)
Potatoes (boiled)
Pumpkin
Squash
Sweet potatoes
Yams

GREEN

VEGETABLES

Alfalfa sprouts
Asparagus
Aubergine
Beans (green/runner)
Bok choy
Broccoli
Brussels sprouts
Cabbage
Capers
Carrots
Cauliflower
Celery
Collard greens
Courgettes
Cucumber
Lettuce

Mangetout
Mushrooms
Mustard greens
Okra
Olives*
Onions
Parsley
Peas
Peppers
Peppers (chilis)
Pickles
Potatoes (new only)
Radicchio
Radishes
Sauerkraut
Scallions
Sugar snap peas
Swiss Chard
Spinach
Tomatoes

*Limit quantity

SERVINGS AND PORTIONS

The G.I. Diet Food Guide makes choosing the right foods for your new eating plan easy. But how much of them should you eat and when? First of all, this isn't a deprivation diet. For the most part, you can have as much of the green-light foods as you like. There are only a few exceptions, which have a higher G.I. rating or calorie content than others. I've listed them along with their recommended serving sizes on the next page.

Some readers have asked me if it's okay to eat twelve apples a day or an entire tub of cottage cheese at a sitting! I don't recommend that you go overboard on quantities of anything. Moderation is key. It's also important that you spread your daily calorie intake evenly throughout the day. If your digestive system is busy processing food and steadily supplying energy to your brain, you won't be looking for

Green-light breads (which have at least 2½ to 3 grams of fibre per slice)	1 slice
Green-light cereals	120g (4oz)
Green-light nuts	8 to 10
Margarine (non-hydrogenated, light)	2 teaspoons
Meat, fish, poultry	120g (4oz) (about the size of a pack of cards)
Olive/rapeseed oil	1 teaspoon
Olives	4 to 5
Pasta	40g (1½oz) uncooked
Potatoes (boiled new)	2 to 3
Rice (basmati, brown, long grain)	50g (1¾oz) uncooked
PHASE II	
Chocolate (70% cocoa)	2 squares
Red wine	1 125ml (5fl oz) glass

high-calorie snacks. I know that many people make a habit of skipping breakfast in the morning, but this is a big mistake. People who miss breakfast leave their stomachs empty from dinner to lunch the next day, often more than sixteen hours! No wonder they overeat at lunch and then look for a sugar fix mid-afternoon as they run out of steam. Always eat three meals – breakfast, lunch and dinner – as well as three snacks – one mid-morning, one mid-afternoon and one before bed – each day. And try to consume approximately the same amount of calories at each principal meal. If you eat a tiny breakfast and then a tiny lunch, you'll feel so hungry by dinner time that you won't be able to stop yourself from overeating.

As well, each meal should contain some vegetables or fruit, some protein and some type of whole grain food. Fruits, vegetables and grains are all carbohydrates, which are the primary source of energy for your body. They are rich in fibre, vitamins and minerals, including antioxidants, which we now believe play a critical role in protecting against disease – especially heart disease and cancer. That's one of the reasons why high-protein diets, which unfortunately have become quite popular in recent years, are so harmful to your long-term health. They prescribe eating a great deal of animal protein, which is high in saturated fat, while severely cutting back on carbohydrates. This causes ketosis, a dangerous electrolyte imbalance and an acid build-up in the blood that can lead to kidney damage, kidney stones and osteoporosis. Side effects include fatigue, headache, nausea, dizziness and bad breath. By minimizing the amount of vegetables, fruits, whole grains and legumes you consume, you deprive your body of essential vitamins and minerals.

With that in mind, vegetables and fruit, most of which are low-calorie and low-G.I., form the base of the G.I. Diet. Now, most offical sources have traditionally suggested that grains should be the largest component of your diet, followed by vegetables and fruit. But by giving grains priority, they are promoting the leading cause of overweight and obesity. Recently, the Mayo Clinic, one of the world's leading medical research centres, has begun to promote vegetables and fruits as the basis of a healthy diet, rather than grains, which is exactly what the G.I. Diet recommends.

Protein is another essential part of your diet. One-half of your dry body weight is made up of protein, i.e., your muscles, organs, skin and hair, and protein is required to build and repair body tissue. It is also much more effective than carbohydrates or fat in satisfying hunger. It acts as a brake in the digestive process and will make you feel fuller longer as well as more alert. So please include some protein in every single meal. Too often we grab a hasty breakfast of coffee and toast – a protein-free meal. Lunch is sometimes not much better: a bowl of pasta with a few slivers of chicken. And a typical afternoon snack of a biscuit, piece of fruit or muffin contains not a gram of protein. Generally, it's not until dinner that we eat protein, usually our entire daily recommended allowance plus some extra. But because protein is a critical brain food, providing amino acids for the neurotransmitters that relay messages in the brain, it would be better to load up on it earlier in the day. That would give you an alert and active mind for your daily activities. The best solution, however, as I've said, is to spread your protein consumption throughout the day to keep you on the ball and feeling full. Choose low-fat proteins such as lean or low-fat meats that have been trimmed of any visible fat; skinless poultry; fresh, frozen or tinned fish (but not the kind that's coated in batter, which is invariably high in fat); shellfish; beans; low-fat dairy products like skimmed milk (believe it or not, after a couple of weeks of drinking it, it tastes just like semi-skimmed), low-fat yoghurt without sugar, and low-fat cottage cheese; egg whites; and tofu.

An easy way to visualize the portion sizes you should be consuming is to imagine your plate divided into three sections. Half the plate should be covered with vegetables and fruit. One of the sources of protein listed above should occupy one quarter of the plate, and the last quarter should be filled with a green-light type of rice, pasta or potato. Below is a diagram of what your green-light dinner plate should look like.

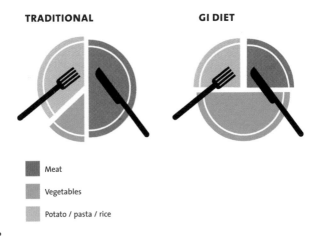

TRADITIONAL

GI DIET

■ Meat

■ Vegetables

■ Potato / pasta / rice

The Most Popular Green-Light Foods

The following is a summary of the most popular green-light foods, which you can look for when shopping.

Almonds
This is the perfect nut in that it has the highest monounsaturated fat (good fat) content of any nut, and recent research indicates that almonds can significantly lower LDL, or bad, cholesterol. They are also excellent sources of Vitamin E, fibre and protein. They provide a great boost to the beneficial fat content of your meals, especially at breakfast or in salads and desserts. Because all nuts are high in calories, use them in moderation.

Apples
A real staple. Eat them fresh for a snack or dessert. Unsweetened apple sauce (e.g. Clearspring Organic Apple Purée) goes well with cereals, or with cottage cheese as a snack.

Barley

An excellent supplement to soups.

Beans

If there's one food you can never get enough of, it's beans, or legumes. This perfect green-light food is high in protein and fibre and can supplement nearly every meal. Make bean salads or just add beans to any salad. Add them to soups, use them to replace some of the meat in casseroles or put them in a meat loaf. You can serve them as a side vegetable or as an alternative to potatoes, rice or pasta. A wide range of tinned and frozen beans is available. Exercise some caution with baked beans, as the sauce can be high-fat and high-calorie. Check labels for low-fat, low-sugar versions and watch the size of your serving. Beans have a well-deserved reputation for creating 'wind', so be patient until your body adapts – as it will – to your increased consumption.

Bread

(See box on page 13). Even with bread made from whole grains, you have to watch your quantity. Have only one slice per meal.

Cereals

Use only large-flake porridge oats, oat bran or other high-fibre cold cereals that have ten grams of fibre or more per serving. Though these cereals are not much fun in themselves, you can liven them up with fruit or fruit-flavoured fat- and sugar-free yoghurt or even sugar-reduced fruit spreads. If you wish to sweeten your cereal, use a sweetener, not sugar.

Cottage cheese

Low-fat or fat-free cottage cheese is an excellent high-protein food. Add fruit to it for a snack or add it to salads.

Eggs

During phase one you should limit your consumption of eggs to no more than half a dozen a week. These should preferably be omega-3 whole eggs because of their heart health benefits. However, you may use as many egg whites as you wish. In phase two you may eat within reason as many eggs as you like unless you have a medical cholesterol problem.

Fish/Shellfish

These are ideal green-light foods, low in fat and cholesterol and a good source of protein. Some coldwater fish such as salmon are also rich in omega-3. Never eat battered or breaded fish.

Food bars

Most food or nutrition bars are dietary disasters, high in carbohydrates and calories but low in protein. These bars are simply quick sugar fixes. There are a few, such as Myoplex or Power Protein

Bars, that have a more equitable distribution of carbohydrates, proteins and fats. Look for 20 to 30 grams of carbohydrates, 12 to 15 grams of protein and 5 grams of fat. This comes to about 220 calories per bar. Keep them at home and at work for a convenient snack – remember that the serving size is half of one bar. In an emergency, it's okay to have one bar plus an apple and a glass of skimmed milk for lunch if you can't get away for a proper break. But try not to make a habit of it.

Grapefruit
One of the top-rated green-light foods. Eat grapefruit as often as you like.

Hamburgers
These are acceptable only if they have been made with extra-lean minced beef that has 10 per cent or less fat. You can add some oat bran to the meat to provide more fibre and less fat. Alternatively, you could use minced turkey or chicken. And

there are some soy substitutes for meat that taste remarkably good and are worth checking out. Keep the serving size at 120g (4oz) and eat open-faced with only half of a wholemeal bun.

Meat
The best green-light meats are skinless chicken and turkey, fully trimmed beef, veal, deli cuts of lean ham, and back bacon. The beef cuts to choose are round, sirloin or tenderloin.

Milk
Use skimmed only. If you have trouble adjusting to it, then use semi-skimmed and slowly wean yourself off it. The fat you're giving up is saturated. Milk is a terrific snack or meal supplement. I drink two glasses of skimmed milk a day, at breakfast and lunch.

Nuts

Nuts are a principal source of 'good' fat, which is essential for your health. Almonds are your best choice. Add them to cereals, salads and desserts. Because they are calorie dense, they must be used in moderation.

Oat bran

You can use this excellent high-fibre food in baking as a partial replacement for flour, or you can make it into a hot cereal.

Oranges

Fresh oranges are excellent as snacks, at breakfast and added to cereals. A glass of orange juice has 2½ times as many calories as a whole orange, so avoid the juice and stick with the real thing.

Pasta

Most pastas are acceptable if you do not overcook them (pasta should be *al dente*, with some firmness to the bite) and if you limit the serving size to a quarter of your plate. Never use pasta as the basis of a meal – it is a side dish only.

Peaches, pears and plums

These fruits are terrific snacks, desserts or additions to breakfast cereal. Buy them fresh, or tinned in water or juice (drain the juice).

Porridge

If you haven't had porridge since you were a kid, now's the time to revisit it. Large-flake, or old-fashioned, porridge is the breakfast of choice, because not only is it green-light, but it also lowers cholesterol. The instant and quick cooking (one-minute) versions are not recommended because they have a far higher G.I. content due to the extra processing of the oats. I like porridge so much, I often have it as a snack with unsweetened apple sauce and sweetener (I use 30g [1oz] oats).

Potatoes
Only boiled new potatoes are acceptable on the G.I. Diet. They have a low starch content, unlike the larger, more mature potatoes, which are very red-light. Still, limit your quantity to two or three per serving.

Rice
Various types of rice have different G.I. ratings, and most of them are red-light. The best kinds are basmati and long grain, and brown is better than white. Don't overcook rice so that it starts to clump together. The more it's cooked, the more glutinous and red-light it becomes.

Soups

Tinned soups have a higher G.I. rating than homemade ones because of the high temperature at which commercial varieties are processed. I have included some brands of tinned soup in the green-light category because these are the best alternative available. Homemade soups are even more green-light.

Sour cream

Low-fat or fat-free sour cream with a little sweetener stirred in is an ideal alternative to whipped cream as a dessert topping. You can also mix fruit or low-sugar fruit spread into it for a creamy dessert.

Soy

Soy protein powder is a simple way to boost the protein level of any meal. It's particularly useful at breakfast for sprinkling over cereal. Look for the kind that has a 90 per cent protein content. It's sometimes labelled 'isolated soy protein powder'. Unflavoured low- or fat-free soya milk is a perfect green-light beverage.

Sweeteners (Sugar Substitutes)

There has been a tremendous amount of misinformation circulating about artificial sweeteners – all of which has been proven groundless. The sugar industry rightly saw these new products as a threat and has done its best to bad-mouth them. You can find an excellent medical overview of sweeteners in the U.S. Food and Drug Administration Consumer Magazine at www.fda.gov. Use, for example, Splenda or Hermesetas Gold to replace sugar in your diet. If you are allergic to sweeteners, then fructose is a better alternative to sugar. The herbal sweetener stevia, which can be found in health food stores, is acceptable if used in moderation since no long-term studies on its usage are available.

Tofu

Though not flavourful in itself, tofu can be spiced up in a variety of ways and is an excellent low-fat source of protein. Use it to boost or replace meat and seafood in stir-fries, burgers and salads.

Yoghurt

Non-fat, fruit-flavoured yoghurt sweetened with aspartame is a great green-light product and has one of the lowest G.I.s of all foods. It makes an ideal snack or a flavourful addition to breakfast cereal or fruit for dessert. I always keep our refrigerator well stocked with a variety of flavours. In fact, my shopping cart is so full of yoghurt containers that fellow shoppers frequently stop me to ask if they are on special!

Yoghurt cheese

A wonderful substitute for sour cream in desserts or in main dishes like chili. Emily has provided a recipe for this green-light staple on page 114 of *Living the Gi Diet*.

Note: Additional updates can be found at **www.gidiet.co.uk.**

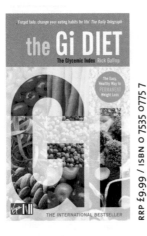
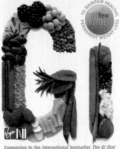